I'm Autistic Get Me Out Of Here!

My Christian Journey on the Autistic Spectrum

By Robert Noble

**Kingdom
Publishers**

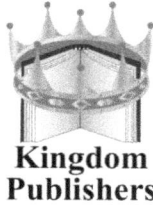

A catalogue record for this book is available from the
British Library.

All Scripture quotations have been taken from the New
International Version of the Bible

ISBN: 978-1-916801-48-6

1st Edition 2025 by Kingdom Publishers, London, UK.

You can purchase copies of this book from any
leading bookstore or at:

www.kingdompublishers.co.uk

Foreword

'I'm Autistic, get me out of here — My Christian life on the Autistic Spectrum — is a very brave and illuminating insight into the real issues facing those with autism today. Robert's enthusiasm is infectious, and his experiences and willingness to share are very touching. His advice will be a great encouragement and source of support to many. I commend this book.'

Rt Revd Sandy Millar, Honorary Assistant Bishop,   Diocese of London
Sandy Millar played a pivotal role in the development and expansion of the Alpha Course as Vicar of Holy Trinity Church Brompton

Robert gives us a very honest, personal and often amusing account of his life on the autistic spectrum. Seeing his form of autism as a gift from God, he invites us to share the ride of his 'slightly quirky, sometimes confusing but ultimately wonderful' and blessed life. A life rooted in the faithfulness and love of God for us all.

Rt Revd Richard Atkinson OBE, Bishop of Bedford

About The Author by Jon Noble

Rob was born in London as the son of a Polish-Jewish tailor in East London. He arrived not long after the end of the Second World War, a few days after the birth of the comedian, Larry David, who has a similar heritage to him. Unlike Larry David, who wants to 'Curb Your Enthusiasm', Rob is full of it!

He grew up in North London, where he spent most of his life. Rob's father arrived in the UK after their Jewish family had to flee from Poland and escape to Canada. They travelled over to England on a ship, where he found his own Christian faith.

Rob's mother descended from the Howe family and his uncle was Sir William Letts, the co-founder of the Automobile Association and a motor industry icon.

There's a saying, 'if you've met one autistic person, you've met one autistic person.' No two are the same. This account of Rob's life shows Rob's story and removes many of the myths about people with autism. One of the misconceptions is that autistic people have no empathy, but Rob shows his great compassion and double empathy for those in the most need.

The book takes you on a journey from Rob's childhood, when he was misunderstood, and society was not accepting or aware of additional needs and how to support these people. These children were labelled as lazy, naughty or stupid. Rob's fascination with furniture and antiques gave him an environment to flourish in.

Acknowledgements

A special thanks to my loving family: my wife Jenny, daughter Clare and son Jonathan, for their constant support through all the ups and downs of my life.

Prayer

Heavenly Father,

In Your infinite wisdom, You have created each of us with unique gifts and challenges. Today, I seek Your guidance and strength as I learn to embrace my autism as a blessing.

Grant me the grace to accept myself fully, knowing that every aspect of my being is a part of Your divine plan. Help me to see the beauty in my differences and to celebrate the strengths that come with my autism. May I find peace in the knowledge that I am wonderfully made in Your image.

Lord, give me the courage to face the difficulties that come my way with resilience and hope. Surround me with love and support and let me be a source of inspiration and strength for others.

As I navigate this journey, teach me to trust in Your purpose for my life. Open my heart to the blessings that come from embracing who I am, and let my life be a testament to Your boundless love and grace.

Amen

Index

Introduction   **11**

Section 1 – My Story   **12**

Chapter 1: Family   12

Chapter 2: An Early Interest in Antiques and Fundraising   14

Chapter 3: Meltdowns, Sensory Overload and New Situations   15

Chapter 4: Stories of Jesus   16

Chapter 5 : My Desire to Raise Money   17

Chapter 6: Challenges at School   18

Chapter 7: Metalwork Class   19

Chapter 8: Mumbling   20

Chapter 9: Beginning My Career   21

Chapter 10: An Emotional Outburst at Work   23

Chapter 11: The Customer is Always Right   24

Chapter 12: Kindness Pays   25

Chapter 13: Changes   26

Chapter 14: Charity Work Continues   28

Chapter 15: Journey to Kenya   29

Chapter 16: My Time in Kenya   30

Chapter 17: My Return to Kenya   32

Chapter 18: Sharing the Peace   33

Chapter 19: Travelling   34

Chapter 20: Love of Animals & Eye Contact   35

Chapter 21: Memory   36

Chapter 22: Understanding Myself   37

Section 2 – Reflection on life and faith   **38**

Chapter 23: Autism in the Context of Faith   38

Chapter 24: Neurodiversity   39

Chapter 25: Visual Thinkers   40

Chapter 26: Stress   41

Chapter 27: Remembering Names   42

Chapter 28: The Importance of Enthusiasm   43

Chapter 29: The Wisdom of Thomas the Tank Engine   44

Chapter 30: The Simple Power of a Smile   45

Chapter 31: The Power of Positive Thinking   46

Chapter 32: Prayer, Faith and Strength   47

Chapter 33: Dyspraxia   48

Chapter 34: Clumsiness   50

Chapter 35: Reflections   51

Chapter 36: Relating Autism to Scripture 1   53

Chapter 37: Relating Autism to Scripture 2   54

Chapter 38: Relating Autism to Scripture 3   55

Chapter 39: Relating Autism to Scripture 4   56

Chapter 40: Relating Autism to Scripture 5   57

Chapter 41: And Finally   58

Introduction

The title of this book describes my struggle to escape from the negative perception of being on the autistic spectrum, and to realise the positive aspects of it that lead to a happy life. I am also dyspraxic and there are two chapters dedicated to this.

This book is a front-row ticket to my roller-coaster ride, complete with unexpected loops, dizzying drops, and —thankfully —a safety harness in the form of my faith. I've gone from the pits of despair to basking in the glorious sunshine of joy, all while navigating life on the autistic spectrum. And let me tell you, it's been quite the adventure. Think less "smooth sailing," and more "trying to ride a unicycle on a tightrope during a windstorm."

With ADHD, OCD, and dyspraxia thrown into the mix, my journey has been like scaling Mount Everest—exhausting, chaotic, but totally worth it. And yes, there have been plenty of metaphorical (and literal) stumbles along the way, but at least I've learned to fall with style.

I know attention spans can be like phone signals— strong one minute, completely gone the next — so I've kept my chapters short and snappy. Feel free to dive in from the start or jump in anywhere like a child in a ball pit.

At the end of the day, I see my form of autism as a gift from God—a slightly quirky, sometimes confusing, but ultimately wonderful blessing. Now, enjoy the ride!

Section 1 – My Story

Chapter 1: Family

I was four when I started to talk. Until I was seven, my autistic response looked like a cross between an enthusiastic bird and Enid Blyton's Noddy. I'd nod my head (with no bell on the top of my hat) or flap my arms as if I were moments away from take-off.

My father was in the RAF for the duration of the Second World War. My brother, who is ten years older than me, barely got to know our dad during those wartime years. Instead, he bonded with our uncle next door, a glazier by trade and, apparently, a stand-in father figure.

When I arrived on the scene, my mum took one look at the situation and made a bold decision: Dad was in charge of me. This meant he got the joy of bath time, bedtime, and all the other glamorous parenting duties.

I grew up in Muswell Hill and living next door were my grandparents, an aunt and uncle and my grandmother's sister. When all nine of us gathered next door, it was less of a cosy get-together and more of a full-blown sensory assault. The noise levels reached were too much for me to bear, and my survival instincts kicked in. My solution? A tactical retreat under the table; my own personal sanctuary of peace and quiet (or at least as much as you can get when surrounded by people above, chatting nineteen to the dozen). Something I disliked was that at mealtimes, my great aunt would ambush me with a giant serviette, tying it around my neck and nearly strangling me (at least, that's how it felt).

We spent a lot of time with them, and I was very uncomfortable with that. Not because they weren't lovely, but because they were far too lovely. I did get some unwelcome attention when we arrived next door, like a hug from my great aunt. I've never been a fan of hugs, and back then, it felt like being trapped in a never-ending cuddle ambush. I however discovered my own escape route, Auntie Dick's house, conveniently located just around the corner. We had affectionate names for each other. I named her "Auntie Dicky Doughnut" and she called me "Mr Oppenheimer". It was a strategic getaway spot, perfect for when I needed a break from my occasionally overwhelming family.

Chapter 2: An Early Interest in Antiques and Fundraising

My lifelong interest in antiques and fundraising started early. As a child, I had a very strong interest in antiques. My great uncle was a famous pioneer in the motor trade and was one of the founders of the AA (the Automobile Association). He lived in a mansion in North Wales, and when we visited, my mother and two aunts used to chat away while Sir William's housekeeper would show me round the house, where I admired his antiques, and loved to see his latest acquisitions.

I loved nothing more than rummaging through jumble sales like a bargain-hunting Indiana Jones. With an eye as sharp as an experienced antique dealer, I would find treasures that turned a profit for Methodist Missions, most of which ended up in the local antique shop right across the street. Fast forward to today, and my obsession has shifted to raising funds for street children. In between I was an active supporter of a children's charity.

Chapter 3: Meltdowns, Sensory Overload and New Situations

Though I was a quiet and shy boy, my behaviour wasn't always impeccable. In fact, my talent for meltdowns persisted well into my early twenties. I remember one particular outburst at age nine when I hurled a wooden clothes hanger through the living room window. My parents, in their infinite patience, gently informed me that my grandpa, a skilled glazier, would sort it out. Clearly, I was a work-in-progress.

Another meltdown came when I was about the same age. My Great-Aunt Rose took me and my mother to Chessington Zoo during the school holidays. It was packed with people, something I could not cope with. I screamed out, "I need to get out of here". This puzzled my mother and aunt.

Starting Sunday School at Muswell Hill Methodist Church was like being tossed into the deep end of a pool without floats. For several weeks I perfected the art of refusing to stay there. Finally, my mum had a brilliant idea and arranged for me to go with someone I knew — a social lifeboat, if you will. This worked wonders, and I managed to make three friends. Our friendship became my sanctuary through the stormy seas of childhood and teenage years.

Chapter 4: Stories of Jesus

When I was seven, Miss Tucker, a retired missionary and my Sunday School teacher with a knack for storytelling, spun tales of her time in China. She was so descriptive that her stories played out in my head.

Miss Tucker spoke about Jesus as if He were her best friend, a lifelong friend she could always count on. I was thrilled to have Jesus as my friend, and feeling His presence gave me a real boost. My favourite "movie repeated in my head" was the one where a group of friends made a hole in the roof and lowered their friend down to Jesus for a miraculous healing. It was like the ultimate DIY project but with divine intervention.

Miss Tucker's stories were so captivating that my mum, at my request, even invited her to lunch. I was eager, not for the food, but for more tales of Jesus, my newfound hero. That was the point when I became a Christian, and throughout my life, in the ups and downs, He has been my close friend. My mind turned those stories into vivid pictures, and my favourite hymn, which I remember clearly, was "Tell Me the Stories of Jesus." As I write this book, I have been a Christian for 70 years!

> Tell me the stories of Jesus
> I love to hear;
> Things I would ask Him to tell me
> If He were here:
> Scenes by the wayside,
> Tales of the sea,
> Stories of Jesus,
> Tell them to me.
>
> *Written in 1885 by William H. Parker*

Chapter 5 : My Desire to Raise Money

I was so influenced by my Sunday School teacher, Miss Tucker, that I developed a burning desire to help children in the poorest parts of the world. So, armed with a trusty notebook, I took on the mission to raise money by regularly collecting from people at the church for the Methodist Missionary Society.

The congregation knew me as the shy boy who would cower if approached. Imagine their shock when I confidently approached them, asking for weekly donations to my cause. Not a single soul turned me down! It was as though they couldn't resist my newfound vocal charm, even though it was through my obsession with making money for my cause.

I even convinced my parents to host coffee mornings at our house, all in aid of mission work. My mum was a sport and went along with it, turning our home into a fundraising hub. I raised and collected money for the Methodist Missionary Society for ten years.

Chapter 6: Challenges at School

My dyspraxia and autism were like a tag-team duo getting me into trouble at school. Teachers punished me for not listening and failing to complete tasks like making craft items. My "abstract art" didn't quite impress. I ended up getting detentions for not paying attention, not finishing the task, and being lazy.

I was a prime target for bullies, both from some classmates and even a few teachers. These incidents often ended in epic meltdowns on my part. One playground saga involved the teacher blowing the whistle, signalling us to stand still like garden gnomes. I complied, but another boy decided to jump on me from behind. Off to the headmaster's office we went! I tried explaining I was innocent to the teacher, but he didn't buy it. I exploded like a volcano, and I remember screaming at him, adding yet another notch to my 'trouble' tally.

I was in my junior school class one day, minding my own business, when I got caught off-guard. We were apparently told to build some kind of robot. Could I do that? Absolutely not. Did that stop me from getting into trouble? Absolutely not. Somehow, I ended up with a detention, but in a spectacular display of my organisational skills, I completely forgot to go. It only hit me when I got home.

The next morning, I dragged myself to school, fully prepared to face my doom. But... nothing. No lecture, no extra punishment. Either my teacher forgot, or I pulled off the greatest accidental escape in detention history. Either way, I wasn't about to question it!

Chapter 7: Metalwork Class

At secondary school I had the *pleasure* of being in a metalwork class, a subject that required precision, coordination, and a general awareness of one's surroundings. Naturally, I was doomed from the start.

Our metalwork teacher was as strict as they come. On day one, he made it very clear, "If anyone leaves the chuck key in the commercial drill, they will receive three lashes of the cane." Message received... well, kind of.

Fast forward a few weeks, and I did exactly what I wasn't supposed to do. I turned on the drill, with the chuck key still inside. What happened next? The key shot out like a missile, zoomed across the room, and embedded itself in the wall opposite.

And then, pure luck struck. The teacher had just stepped out of the room. He didn't see a thing. I stood there, frozen, waiting for someone to rat on me. But miraculously, my classmates stayed silent. No one said a word. I don't know if it was loyalty or sheer amusement at my near-death experience, but I was *very* grateful.

Lesson learned? Power tools and I should probably never be in the same room.

Chapter 8: Mumbling

I'm more comfortable addressing an entire crowd than chatting with just one person or a small group. But throw me into a circle where I have to introduce myself, and I find that even harder.

I was seventeen, and for the first time, I went on holiday alone to a Methodist Guild Holiday. Tradition dictated that everyone should sit in a circle and take turns saying their name, where they were from, and their job. Cue the nerves.

At the time, I worked for an estate agent. When it was my turn, I nervously mumbled my name, where I was from, and what I did for a living. The host, not hearing me, asked, "What does that involve?" I mumbled again, "Letting offices." Cue the puzzled looks.

Later, someone came up to me and said, "I'm surprised you came to a Christian holiday working for a betting office!" Other people there gave me strange looks. That's when I realised my mumbling had led them to think I was promoting gambling instead of property!

For those of us on the autism spectrum, these moments of social anxiety can be all too relatable. We might not always get it right, but at least we provide some memorable moments!

Chapter 9: Beginning My Career

I left school at seventeen. After six months working for an estate agent, I got a job with Maples, the furniture store. I stayed there for five years but was disappointed to find no vacancies in their antique department.

In 1971 I secured a job based in the antique department of another London department store, where I was based for ten years. I was able to sell anywhere in the whole of the furniture department. Some rich customers let me furnish their property, allowing me to choose what I thought they would like. Two customers even trusted me with their store credit card.

One rich Arab customer arrived to meet me in the store first thing in the morning. He had his son arriving the next morning. An empty London flat was ready for him and I was to furnish it with everything, that very day. It was like the TV game "Supermarket Sweep" with me rushing round the various departments getting everything from sofas to can openers and arranging a van to take them to the flat. I am sure it was my hyper-focus that helped me achieve this task.

My drawing skills leave much to be desired, my real talent lies in visually and instinctively knowing what people like. I threw myself into designing room layouts during my time at the store. I had this knack for instinctively knowing what to recommend for the clients I interacted with.

When I later landed a job as a buyer for a top London store in 1981, my senses kicked in again. I could just tell what people wanted. I'd visit suppliers, and while their reps tried to sell me something, I was busy flipping through possible covers and vividly imagining the sofa and chairs in a perfect room setting, ignoring what the seller said. It was like playing furniture Tetris in my head.

All of us on the spectrum have God-given talents, and mine just happens to be visualising and knowing people's tastes

Chapter 10: An Emotional Outburst at Work

An example of me losing control, which surprisingly had a happy ending, took place at the store where I worked. I was passing through the games department when I overheard a sales assistant telling a customer, "It really does work; I've had messages from my grandma and great aunt." I turned around and saw she was trying to sell a Ouija board.

I went into an uncontrollable strop and shouted at her, "I can't believe what you are saying!" and stormed off. I expected some serious repercussions for my outburst. Not knowing the gift buyer, I went to the hardware buyer, whom I knew from one of the churches in Barnet where I lived, and told him what happened. An hour later I received the news that all the Ouija boards had been taken off sale.

Chapter 11: The Customer is Always Right

Something I was taught is "The customer is always right" but anyone who is in retail knows this is often not correct. I have lost my cool with customers a few times. Here are a couple of examples. A customer was walking her dog in the furniture department where I worked, and I noticed it cocked its leg up to a very expensive sofa and urinated. I exploded when I saw what had happened and inappropriately gave the woman a piece of my mind! Another incident was when I once completely lost it with royalty. Not our late British Queen Mother but a Queen Mother from a far-off land, complete with an entourage, an attitude, and apparently, zero concept of the word "no."

I was showing Her Royal Highness around the antiques department when she laid eyes on a stunning screen—truly fit for a palace. She pointed at it and declared, *"I want."* Not "How much?" or *"*Tell me more,*"* just a regal command as if she was ordering room service.

I gently informed her that, unfortunately, the screen was already sold to another customer. That's when things took a turn. She didn't just offer to buy it—she offered me a personal bonus on top of the price to make it *disappear* into her entourage's hands, as if I was running a black-market antique smuggling ring on the side.

I politely (but firmly) said, "No." And that's when *she* lost the plot. I, in true customer service solidarity, followed suit. There we were: two grown adults in a standoff over a folding screen, arguing like toddlers over a toy neither of us technically owned.

She wouldn't give up, and honestly, looking back, I realised that she probably hadn't heard the word "no" her whole life. In her world, saying "no" to her was unheard of and she just could not cope with it.

Chapter 12: Kindness Pays

Back in the late 1970s a fabulously wealthy lady, draped in designer everything and probably wearing perfume worth more than my monthly wage, approached me looking for the lift to the perfumery department. I offered to escort her there, like some kind of department store butler.

When we arrived, she looked at me, gave a gracious "Thank you," and handed me a crisp £5 note. Now, that might not sound impressive today, but back then that was about £30 in today's money and a ticket to instant staff room celebrity status. I half-expected the other assistants to lift me onto their shoulders and chant my name.

On the flip side, in the very same store, I had a regular visitor: a sweet elderly lady who was always "looking for a small tea table." Truth be told, really she was just looking for someone to talk to, and I was happy to play the part of furniture tour guide and occasional therapist.

We'd wander through the furniture department together, nodding thoughtfully at tables she had absolutely no intention of buying. Like many local widows, she was simply lonely, and if a stroll past the mahogany section helped her feel seen and heard, I was more than glad to oblige.

Sometimes, kindness comes with a fiver. Other times, it comes with a smile and a story. Both, as it turns out, are pretty priceless.

On another occasion, I was on the way back to my department, and a shabbily dressed couple approached me, saying nobody would serve them. I said I would gladly help. It turned out they were funfair owners and spent a fortune! Well, you should have seen some of my colleagues' faces.

Chapter 13: Changes

My close-knit friendship with the three boys from Sunday School continued into our early 20s. Then life changed for the worse: Malcolm tragically passed away from cancer, Richard became an Aussie adventurer, and Brian got hitched and moved far away.

The following years were tough. I became depressed, with my records as my constant companions. The highlight of my week was Sunday, thanks to the church's 20+ club.

Life changed for me with the help of a young man called Roger. During the January sale at the London store in 1974, I found myself on the furniture floor, surrounded by 29 other salespeople all vying for commissions, like seagulls fighting over a single chip. Each of us was given an assistant and mine was Roger, a university student in his final year, with dreams of becoming a training manager. For a month he worked with me, offering support and encouragement.

Though technically I was the one training Roger, there ended up being an amusing role reversal. To his credit, Roger listened intently, nodded in all the right places, and took everything in like a sponge. It was almost as if he was studying me instead of furniture sales.

Roger took one look at me clinging to the bottom of the sales chart like a limpet, noticed I was too shy to actually approach customers, and decided it was time for an intervention. He clocked my nerves from a mile away and, in his infinite wisdom, suggested I enrol in a Dale Carnegie course called "Effective Speaking and Human Relations", which I did, and it did wonders for my confidence. The real breakthrough, however, came when Roger tapped into my love of acting. "Think of the Antique department as your stage," he said, "and you're the lead actor. The customers? Just fellow cast members waiting for you to engage." Suddenly, selling didn't feel like a nerve-wracking sales pitch, it was a performance! And let me tell you, once I stepped into my role, my sales skyrocketed. Turns out, I wasn't bad at selling after all—I just needed the right script!

The following December, in 1975, I met Jenny at the church 20+ club, the girl of my dreams. In October 1976, we were married: I don't like to hang around! This began a new, brighter chapter in my life; later, going on to have our two children. We now have five grandchildren, as well as a son- and daughter-in-law, bringing us much joy and fun.

Chapter 14: Charity Work Continues

For the next twenty years I served on the committee of The Barnet and Finchley 'Save The Children' Fund. I organised a variety of events such as quizzes, auctions, stalls at local fairs, music events, and auctions of promises. I also released two singles with the help of the young people's groups I was involved with as a youth leader.

One single was called "Save the Children," sung by Dave Pearson. The record made money for Save the Children. Sadly, Dave died suddenly at the young age of 37.

 Back in 1986 I was connected to a group of boys in Mozambique who had been kidnapped by the Renamo and forced to become soldiers. Renamo (Resistência Nacional Moçambicana) was a rebel group in Mozambique that used child soldiers during the brutal civil war (1977–1992). Thousands of children were forcibly recruited, often abducted from their villages, and subjected to extreme violence to break their will. They were trained to fight, forced to commit atrocities, and used as frontline soldiers, porters, or spies. When rescued by government troops, they went to a special centre where producing music helped them heal.

I arranged for three boys in a youth group I was involved with to link up with the boys in Mozambique and exchange music tapes. Our youth club boys recorded a rap called "Mozambique," which became a great hit in Mozambique and was played frequently on the radio there. Organising and planning events has been a great way for me to channel my energy and passion.

For the last 10 years, since I have been in Haslemere, I have sold greetings cards and fair trade carvings in aid of my street children's charities.

Chapter 15: Journey to Kenya

In 1997, a pastor from Kenya visited the church I was attending. He came armed with some beautiful pictures from his congregation, hoping to sell them. Coincidentally, The Stable, a local church, was hosting an art exhibition featuring local talent. I thought, "Why not add a few more paintings to the mix?" So, I asked if I could include the pictures Pastor John had brought along, and they said yes. The pictures sold well. The pastor then invited me to visit Kenya. Naturally, I said yes, because who could resist the chance to see the world from a completely different perspective?

Later that year I found myself travelling to Kenya to stay with Pastor John. I was sitting next to a Kenyan who had been visiting support churches in the UK, and we were chatting away. It was announced that at Nairobi Airport a plane was stuck on the runway, and we could not land. Mombasa Airport was fully booked. An announcement was made that the pilot was seeking somewhere else to land. Half an hour passed, and we heard nothing.

The Kenyan pastor whom I had been talking to said, "Join me at the front of the plane". I instinctively followed him to the front. He led a prayer and asked God to find a slot for us. We remained at the front while people on the plane took it in. Everyone had been very worried. Within 30 seconds, an announcement told us we were to land in Madagascar. The whole plane clapped and cheered as we returned to our seats. There was a great opportunity to witness during the flight.

Chapter 16: My Time in Kenya

Arriving in Kenya was an exhilarating experience. The people were so happy, genuinely happy, despite living in poverty. It was as if they had discovered the secret to life that most of us miss in our quest for more stuff. Their simple way of living was surprisingly refreshing. Yes, they faced hardships, like not having access to clean water, but their resilience was truly inspiring.

And as for me? Well, I had the joy of waking up with the sunrise, witnessing Pastor John's wife cooking meals over three stones. The next day we went on a mission to feed the street children in Naivasha. I was shocked and amazed to hear about the street children, how they were abused and treated so badly and went hungry.

When we got there, the children were very receptive; they were very polite. There was one boy who was a bit concerned because his friend wasn't there, so the people I was with allowed him to go and find him so he could share in the food as well.

We also saw a boy in a different part of town on his own. He seemed traumatised and very young. The local person in charge of the programme explained that the boy could not talk and showed no reaction when people spoke to him. We gave him some food, which he ate so fast it was as if he had never eaten before. He looked at me, and in his eyes I saw the eyes of Jesus, and I made the decision for the rest of my life to go and help the street children in any way I could. I now look back and wonder if that boy was autistic. Having done the research, I have found out that many of the autistic children in Kenya are given no help at all.

When I returned to England, I was on a mission—determined to help the amazing people I had met in Kenya. One of them was a remarkable woman named Catherine, who was tirelessly caring for children. She needed a dormitory for the boys in her care, and I thought, "Well, if I can get a group of people to buy into this, we might just have a chance." So, I returned to Barnet, rallied the troops at The Methodist Church and within two months we had raised enough money to make Catherine's dream a reality.

Sadly, Catherine passed away a few years ago due to COVID-19. She was an incredible person and is greatly missed. The Neema Children's Home is still thriving, and I have been privileged to help them over the years.

Recently, I heard about a 10-year-old autistic boy in Kenya who has a single-parent mum who works long hours to make a living. The wages are barely enough to live on. Her son Levis needs to be locked in the house all day when she is working, which is very traumatic for him. I decided I would pay the fees to send him to a special school that caters for those who are autistic. Now, the Pangani School where he attends receives support from The Neema Society.

Chapter 17: My Return to Kenya

On my second trip to Kenya I lugged along a computer and printer to help the Pastor's church and community. Approaching customs at Nairobi Airport, I braced myself for what I imagined would be a great expense to bring them through customs. I prayed fervently, hoping for divine intervention.

Sure enough, my prayers were answered in the form of a cheerful, Christian customs officer. He not only let me through without a hitch but also applauded my efforts.

Upon arriving at the church, I discovered a minor hiccup; the promised electrical supply was absent. The next morning, I marched into the local office that supplies the power, with the Pastor, and had a 'friendly chat' with the manager. Miraculously, by the end of the afternoon, the electricity was flowing, and so was my relief.

The downside of all of this was the trauma of seeing so much suffering caused me a lot of stress, resulting in me being unwell for some time. However, looking back, it was God who used it for His purpose, and I would not want it any other way.

Chapter 18: Sharing the Peace

In 2015 we moved to Haslemere and started to worship at St. Stephen's Church, a friendly place with a lively modern service that we enjoyed. However, I do find one aspect challenging: the predominantly Anglican way of sharing the peace during communion. It is an embarrassing situation for me, as I become acutely aware of anyone coming towards me and dread any physical contact.

One incident stands out: while not noticing a lady coming towards me during the peace-sharing, she suddenly turned to embrace me. Startled, I jumped aside, narrowly avoiding her hug. It was embarrassing, and I apologised to her. I usually put my arm out at full length for a straightforward handshake.

The worst scenario when talking to someone — and I'm sure you know exactly what I mean — is when someone gets way too close while talking to me. I take a step back, and they take a step forward like it's some sort of unwanted tango. At that point, I have two options: keep stepping back until I eventually reach the wall of where I am or politely let them know that personal space is a thing, and I'd prefer to keep mine intact!

Chapter 19: Travelling

I get stressed if my routine changes—even a little. Just the thought of a disruption sends me into a mild panic. Take holidays, for instance. The lead-up to them is the stuff of nightmares. Our daughter works with a Bible Translation organisation in Papua New Guinea, which means a trip involving four planes and nearly three days of travel. Yes, three days. That's not a journey; that's a saga.

When we finally land in Port Moresby, I feel like I've won a small victory. I can almost hear the angels singing as we recover from our jetlag at the Holiday Inn. Nothing quite like a hotel bed to make you forget you've just spent an eternity in the air. But it's not over yet! We then take a small plane to Ukarumpa, where the family lives. I have to admit, the small plane bit always makes me a bit twitchy. As we leave Port Moresby the pilot always prays for a safe flight before we take off. I find that very comforting.

However, once we get there, it's like entering a different world—peaceful, welcoming, and surrounded by Christians from all over the globe. It's the perfect spot for someone like me who appreciates a bit of tranquillity. Honestly, after all that travel chaos I find Ukarumpa surprisingly calm. It suits me perfectly—there, I can actually breathe again.

Chapter 20: Love of Animals & Eye Contact

Every Friday afternoon I attend the Cats Protection premises and socialise with cats. The majority of them are most welcoming and I enjoy their company. They are very friendly and relaxing to be with. Each one has their own personality and behaves in their own special way. I would recommend anyone on the autistic spectrum to get a pet or, like me, to go to Cats Protection or similar.

I have noticed that some cats I visit make eye contact and others do not. It is the same with people. Many on the autistic spectrum avoid eye contact. I found making eye contact was not easy to do, but something I learnt when made aware how important it was to do this.

Chapter 21: Memory

At 77, my short-term memory is... let's just say it's gone on a bit of an extended tea break. But my long-term memory? Oh, that's still firing on all cylinders.

I can't remember what I had for breakfast yesterday, but I *do* remember crystal-clear details from decades ago. For example, my very first retail job: I can tell you that in 1968, a reproduction mahogany bureau—stock number V513, no less—was priced at exactly £59. Not £60, not £58... *£59*. That's the kind of deeply useless knowledge I have, with my brain being wired differently from that of most people.

Chapter 22: Understanding Myself

After reading a few books, I noticed that I could identify with several autistic and ADHD traits. I also had some helpful discussions with my GP about these conditions. Discovering that I have ADHD was oddly comforting and answered questions I had no answers to during my earlier life. I realised I wasn't alone in my zany adventures. It's a bit like finding out there's a whole club of people whose lives are affected by it. But listen, at least we're in it together. Although it is not possible for the challenges to magically disappear, it is certainly possible to reduce the stress that comes with them.

Section 2 – Reflection on life and faith

Chapter 23: Autism in the Context of Faith

To understand autism through the lens of faith, we need to start with the basics: love, acceptance and inclusion. After all, Christianity isn't about ticking boxes or fitting neatly into social circles. It's about seeing the God-given worth in every person, labels or no labels.

The church has a golden opportunity to practise what it preaches by making people with autism feel valued, understood, and, most importantly, not like some sort of divine admin error. By embracing these differences, the faith community doesn't just help autistic individuals, it enriches itself, gaining a deeper appreciation for the wonderfully diverse ways God has designed us.

Thankfully, I've found that my own church — St Stephen's Church, Shottermill — has nailed this beautifully. The congregation has embraced all the above with open arms, and not just in a polite, tea-and-biscuits sort of way, but in a genuine, Christ-like fashion. It turns out that when a church truly reflects God's love, there's room for everyone, quirks and all.

Chapter 24: Neurodiversity

Autism Spectrum Disorder (ASD) affects the way people communicate, interact, and generally navigate the social world, which — let's be honest — can be a minefield at the best of times. In faith communities, where unspoken social rules and traditions often reign supreme, this can lead to a few misunderstandings. Suddenly, an autistic person's honest remark during a sermon, or preference for a quiet corner over coffee and mingling, is seen as "odd" rather than simply *different*.

The result? Christians with autism can sometimes feel like they're on the outside looking in, like being invited to a dance but not quite knowing the steps. However, with a bit of personalised support, a splash of education, and the revolutionary idea of simply talking to people (rather than making assumptions), churches can become places where neurodiversity isn't just *tolerated* but *celebrated*. After all, God created us all uniquely, and let's be honest, if He wanted everyone to be the same, he wouldn't have given us such wonderfully varied brains.

Embracing neurodiversity doesn't just help autistic individuals; it enriches the entire faith community. If that means rethinking the usual post-service chit-chat protocol or being a little more flexible with traditions, well, surely that's a small price to pay for a more inclusive and loving church!

Chapter 25: Visual Thinkers

Stories appear like movies in my head. I'm a visual thinker. I just wish I had the artistic talent to go with it, especially coming from a family of artists. Sadly, my stick figures still look like they've had a rough day.

Some autistic people have amazing abilities. Temple Grandin talks about her own visual thinking experiences in her book "Temple Grandin: How the Girl Who Loved Cows Embraced Autism and Changed the World." She invented things in her mind to help make farming more humane for cattle. Temple was born a month after me and, like me, she wasn't talking at four years old. The authorities pushed to get Temple into an institution, expecting her to stay there for the rest of her life. However, her mother gave her the care and attention that led her to be very successful. I guess we both took the scenic route to speech.

Stephen Wiltshire, MBE (born 24 April 1974) is a British architectural artist and certified genius. He can draw an entire landscape from memory after seeing it just once. After flying over London, he came back to his studio and drew the cityscape in jaw-dropping detail. Meanwhile, I struggle trying to draw a decent circle.

Chapter 26: Stress

Stress affects each of us differently. For me, it can feel like an emotional volcano just beneath the surface, ready to erupt. Over time, I've learned to recognise the warning signs and take steps to manage them. Prayer has been a lifeline—talking to God, experiencing the comfort of the Holy Spirit, and knowing I'm not facing my struggles alone brings me peace. Alongside that, physical activity, country walks and cycling , have also been incredibly helpful.

Sometimes, when I'm deeply absorbed in something I'm passionate about, it's genuinely difficult, and even stressful, to shift my focus, especially when I'm asked to turn my attention to something more urgent. I realise this can sometimes appear as if I'm disinterested in the request or the person making it, but that's never my intention. I know this can be hurtful, especially to those close to me, like my family. Understanding that this reaction is part of how my autism affects me, I've been working hard to become more aware of these moments and to gently redirect myself when needed.

If you're also on the autism spectrum and this sounds familiar, I encourage you to make a conscious effort to be aware of those around you. It's not always easy, but small steps can make a big difference—for both you and the people who care about you.

Chapter 27: Remembering Names

It is important to take the trouble to remember people's names. Addressing people by their name will mean a lot to them. Lord Tonypandy (George Thomas) met my mother once at a garden event at Muswell Hill Methodist Church. He was introduced by my Aunt Marjory, who knew him, and she simply said, "This is my sister, Eddy." A few years later my mother met him in a lift at St Thomas's Hospital. He turned to her and said, "Hello, Eddy, how is your sister Marjory these days?" What an incredible man was he to remember my mother like he did.

Chapter 28: The Importance of Enthusiasm

A vital message in this book is to be enthusiastic in everything you do. Especially for those on the autistic spectrum, it can be a helpful bridge to connect with the world.

Start your day with a burst of enthusiasm, even on a Monday morning (yes, even then). Is there a chore you've been dodging for ages? Grab it by the horns with enthusiasm. Have an idea you want to pitch to your boss? Deliver it with a double dose of enthusiasm.

In the Bible, the closest word to enthusiasm is "zealous" so go ahead, channel your inner zealot!

Chapter 29: The Wisdom of Thomas the Tank Engine

"Thomas the Tank Engine" is a beloved book and TV programme that is enjoyed by both children and adults alike. It teaches determination, which is a valuable lesson for people of all ages. Phrases such as, "I'm sure I can, I know I can " send a message of positive thinking, while "Little engines can do big things" and "We're all useful, no matter what size we are" are encouraging messages.

In the case of failure, it reminds us that "Sometimes you have to go backwards to go forwards." If things don't go as planned, there is no shame in starting from the beginning. The story also emphasises that "There's no harm in asking for help."

Chapter 30: The Simple Power of a Smile

A smile is a beautiful gift from God, a silent expression of joy and love that reflects His grace. It's like a warm light shining through the soul, offering comfort and encouragement to those around us.

A smile has the power to heal, to uplift, and to remind us of God's ever-present love. It's a reminder that no matter the trials we face, there's always hope, always a reason to rejoice in His goodness. Just as Jesus showed His love through His actions, a simple smile can be a reflection of His heart; gentle, kind, and full of compassion. When we smile, we share a little bit of God's light with the world, spreading warmth and peace in the way only He can inspire.

Chapter 31: The Power of Positive Thinking

If you think you are beaten, you are;
If you think you dare not, you don't.
If you like to win, but you think you can't,
It is almost certain you won't.

If you think you'll lose, you're lost.
For out in the world we find
Success begins with a fellow's will;
It's all in the state of mind.

If you think you are outclassed, you are;
You've got to think high to rise.
You've got to be sure of yourself before
You can ever win a prize.

Life's battles don't always go
To the stronger or faster man.
But soon or late the man who wins
Is the man WHO THINKS HE CAN!

Written in 1920 by Walter D. Wintle.
(The capitalisation is my own)

Chapter 32: Prayer, Faith and Strength

Psalm 27:1: "The Lord is my light and my salvation—whom shall I fear?" reminds us that no matter the struggles we face, we are never alone. And 2 Corinthians 4:16-18 encourages us to look beyond our present challenges, knowing that our inward strength is being renewed day by day.

Prayer looks different for everyone, especially for those on the autism spectrum. Through my faith journey, I've found prayer methods that bring me peace and help me connect with God in ways that feel natural to me. One way is by seeking the Holy Spirit to power my daily life.

While group prayer can sometimes feel overwhelming, being part of a supportive church community has been meaningful for me. Small prayer groups or discussions allow me to share and listen to others without feeling pressured. These prayer practices have helped me grow spiritually and connect with God in my own way. By sharing them, I hope to encourage others, both autistic individuals and those who support them, to explore different prayer methods that suit their needs. A more inclusive approach to prayer can help churches become spaces where everyone can thrive in their faith.

Chapter 33: Dyspraxia

I think the best way to describe dyspraxia is 'living in a whirlwind of chaos'. It is a condition that affects motor skills and coordination; I've mastered the art of complicating simple tasks. Tying shoelaces remains a mystery; Velcro shoes solve my problem now. Buttons, clasps, and traditional can-openers can be part of a daily challenge, and DIY projects tend to end with abstract wall damage. The room I once attempted to wallpaper and paint? It still hasn't forgiven me.

At our last house, our next-door neighbour was so dismayed when he saw how messy our garage was that he marked every shelf and drawer with labels to help me find things.

As a child, sports were an uphill struggle. I was always the last to be picked for football teams. Later, as a youth club leader, I unintentionally became a source of entertainment, spectacularly failing at ice-skating and struggling to even hit the golf ball, much to the amusement of the children. As part of my charity work, I was once conducting an auction. So that everyone could see me, I stood on a window ledge. In the excitement, I lost my balance and fell straight on my face – going, going gone! The story was reported in The Sunday Mirror.

I can even use my dyspraxia to make my grandchildren laugh. I recently set up a prank with a rubber egg, which I inserted in an egg box, ready to throw at my grandson. When the moment came for the joke, I picked the wrong egg out of the carton and threw it towards him onto the floor. Rather than the expected bounce, there was a loud crack. Needless to say, I had egg on my face!

Eating is another adventure. I'm a "generous eater", gifting crumbs and spills to everyone nearby.

People who are not familiar with dyspraxia may perceive us as unintelligent. This can be frustrating, because the only thing worse than struggling to perform these tasks is being judged by others. I hesitate to use the word stupid, but let's face it: many people who are unaware of our condition tend to think that we're a bit thick.

Chapter 34: Clumsiness

Clumsiness is a speciality of mine, and I've mastered the art of complicating simple tasks. Dropping things, bumping into things, being unable to knock a nail in the wall straight are examples of this.

When asking for directions I have great difficulty with the response people give. When someone says, "Turn left, then take the second right." I'm already lost. Now, without Google Maps, I'd probably wander into another country. My sense of balance has been a lifelong challenge, resulting in more encounters with the ground than I care to admit. Thankfully, a balance course six years ago brought noticeable improvement.

Being dyspraxic and on the spectrum means my conversations can be a bit confused. Sometimes I struggle to articulate my thoughts, or I misinterpret what others say, leading to misunderstandings. This means my conversations can feel like a high-stakes round of broken telephone, except I'm both the sender and receiver, and neither of us knows what's going on. I either can't find the right words, or I misinterpret what's being said, leading to moments of pure, unintentional comedy. Thankfully, my wife is fluent in "Me" and can usually untangle my verbal spaghetti.

Chapter 35: Reflections

I like to think of myself as recognising musical talent. While I never mastered the art of playing an instrument (my attempts at the piano were particularly harrowing with my music teacher telling my mother I was a lost cause), I've always had an uncanny knack for recognising musical brilliance.

Back in the day, there was a TV show called "Juke Box Jury", where new pop songs were rated from one to five. I consistently gave fives to tracks that others dismissed.

Take my schoolmate Dave Davies, for instance. He used to perform at our Methodist youth club with his brother Sir Ray Davies and others including Peter Quaife (who incidentally was a pupil in my aunt's Sunday school class) guitar in hand, strumming away. I remember thinking, " This group — the Ravens — are something special." Next thing you know, they changed their name to The Kinks and became one of the most iconic bands of the '60s.

Then there was young Simon Nicol, a doctor's son who frequented our youth gatherings. His guitar skills were evident even then. He often used to sing and play the guitar at the same youth club. I had a hunch he'd make it big, and lo and behold, he went on to form Fairport Convention, a cornerstone of British folk rock.

If I were asked who were the three people who fired me up for Jesus during my life it would be:

1.   My Sunday School teacher, Miss Tucker

2.   Sandy Millar, who came over to the store where I worked from Holy Trinity, Brompton and led the Christian fellowship

3.   And — fast forward to this century — a young man named Jack Robson*, from my St Stephen's home group.

All three have had a great influence and increased my enthusiasm for Jesus.

Jack Robson is an exceptionally gifted Christian singer and songwriter whose music reflects both heartfelt faith and artistic depth. His lyrics are honest, soul-stirring, and rooted in a genuine love for Jesus, offering encouragement, challenge, and comfort in equal measure.

Whether you're going through a difficult season or simply need a reminder of God's presence, Jack's songs have a way of meeting you where you are. I wholeheartedly encourage you to look him up on Spotify and YouTube. Take the time to listen.

Jack has also produced a recording of a song I composed called "I Think You Know" for The Neema Society, recorded by Woolly Hat Studios, Haslemere.

Chapter 36: Relating Autism to Scripture 1

John 15:4 *"Remain in me. As I also remain in you. No branch can bear fruit by itself; It must remain in the vine. Neither can you bear fruit unless you remain in me."*

People with autism may connect with others in different ways, but each way is just as important. Like a branch getting strength from a vine, they need support, understanding, and a sense of belonging to thrive. Building these connections can take patience and empathy, but they help bring out each person's unique strengths.

Autism is a spectrum, so everyone's experiences are different. But one thing stays the same, connection matters. Whether through family, friends, support groups, or faith, staying connected helps them grow, stay strong, and share their unique gifts with the world. Remember, remaining with Jesus at all times is so important.

Chapter 37: Relating Autism to Scripture 2

Philippians 4:13 *"I can do all this through him who gives me strength."*

Whether navigating social interactions, sensory sensitivities, or personal milestones, His strength is my constant support. I am resilient, capable, and beautifully unique, and with His unwavering strength, I can achieve great things and overcome any obstacle.

This reflects the idea that individuals with autism have unique strengths and challenges and with faith and support, they can accomplish incredible feats and navigate their journey with courage.

Chapter 38: Relating Autism to Scripture 3

Psalm 27:1 *"The Lord is my light and my salvation—whom shall I fear? The Lord is the stronghold of my life—of whom shall I be afraid?"*

For individuals on the autism spectrum, the world can sometimes feel overwhelming—full of uncertainty, sensory challenges, and social difficulties. Loud noises, social situations, and changes can bring anxiety, but this verse reminds us that God is a source of light and strength. Just as light helps us see clearly in the dark, God provides guidance and comfort in moments of confusion or fear.

Autistic individuals may face challenges that make them feel different or isolated, but they are not alone. God's presence is a constant source of reassurance, offering stability when things feel uncertain. No matter how difficult the journey may be, God's love and strength provide a safe foundation to rely on.

This verse encourages not just those with autism, but everyone, to find confidence in God's protection. With Him as our stronghold, we can face the world without fear, knowing that we are deeply valued and never alone.

Chapter 39: Relating Autism to Scripture 4

1 Peter 5:7 *"Cast all your anxiety on Him because He cares for you."*

This verse reminds us that we don't have to carry our worries alone. God understands our struggles and wants to help.

No matter how hard things feel, we can trust that God is always there, offering comfort and peace. He cares for each of us, just as we are.

Chapter 40: Relating Autism to Scripture 5

2 Corinthians 4:16-18 *"Therefore we do not lose heart. Though outwardly we are wasting away, yet inwardly we are being renewed day by day. For our light and momentary troubles are achieving for us an eternal glory that far outweighs them all. So we fix our eyes not on what is seen, but on what is unseen, since what is seen is temporary, but what is unseen is eternal."*

This Corinthians passage reminds us to stay strong and hopeful even when life is tough. It tells us that even if we feel as if we're struggling on the outside, we are growing and getting better on the inside every day. These small and temporary problems are helping us prepare for a future that is much better. We should focus on the good things that aren't always visible, rather than just the problems we see now.

When thinking about autism, this message applies well. Autism can bring unique challenges for both those with the condition and their families. However, the scripture encourages us to look beyond the struggles and see the inner strengths and potential of each person with autism. Although there may be difficulties, there is also inner growth, renewal and a journey towards greater understanding and acceptance. For many individuals with autism, the journey may include tough moments but also amazing abilities and perspectives that are not always obvious. These temporary challenges can lead to significant personal growth and the development of unique talents that greatly benefit society.

Chapter 41: And Finally

No matter the obstacles, whether physical, social, or emotional, we all have unique strengths to offer. For those with autism, these strengths can shine brightly when given the support and understanding they need to flourish. Their presence provides strength at all times. By putting our faith in Him we can navigate our journey and achieve great things.

Thank you for reading my book, I hope you have found it interesting.

Please take time to visit my website for the latest information.
www.theneemasociety.com

The Neema Society QR code

All the profit made from the sale of this book will be paid to
Footsteps International, to support the needs of street children in
Kenya and also Pangani Special School, an educational institution
dedicated to supporting children with Autism and those with special
needs.

Footsteps International

Save The Children   Singer: Dave Pearson

I Think You Know Singer: Jack Robson

Jack Robson on Spotify

www.ingramcontent.com/pod-product-compliance
Ingram Content Group UK Ltd.
Pitfield, Milton Keynes, MK11 3LW, UK
UKHW050915240925
8053UKWH00053B/1252

9 781916 801486